WORKOUT LOG

COVER ART CREATED BY FREEPIK
INSIDE ART BY FREEPIK

ISBN-13: 978-1975887162
ISBN-10: 1975887166

IF YOU WANT TO TAKE YOUR WORKOUT TO THE NEXT LEVEL YOU HAVE TO GET INTO A HABIT OF RECORDING EVERYTHING.

INSIDE THIS BOOK YOU WILL FIND A SPACE TO RECORD YOUR DAILY WORKOUT. YOU HAVE SPACE TO RECORD 10 EXERCISES A DAY AND 6 SETS. DON'T FEEL LIKE YOU HAVE TO USE ALL OF THE SPACE, BUT IF YOU NEED MORE JUST GO TO THE NEXT DAYS LOG AND CONTINUE IT THERE.

ALONG WITH YOUR WORKOUT LOGS YOU'LL FIND SPACE TO RECORD YOUR MEASUREMENTS AND FOOD (CALORIE, FAT, CARBS) INTAKE FOR A YEAR.

THIS BOOK IS NOT INTENDED TO GIVE WORKOUT ADVICE ONLY TO GIVE YOU A SPACE TO RECORD WHAT YOU CHOSE TO DO. USE IT HOWEVER FITS BEST FOR YOU.

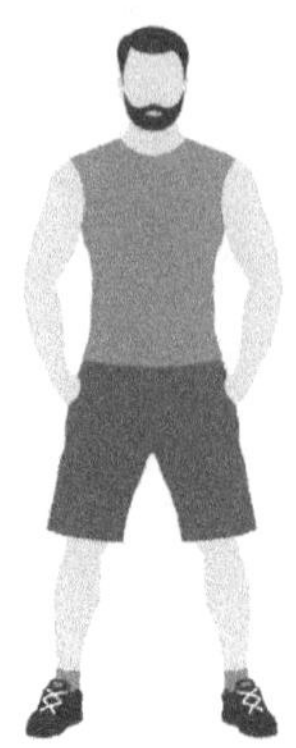

BODY MEASUREMENTS

	DATE:________	DATE:________	DATE:________	DATE:________
WEIGHT				
NECK				
SHOULDERS				
CHEST				
BICEP (L)				
BICEP (R)				
WAIST				
HIPS				
THIGH (L)				
THIGH (R)				
CALF (L)				
CALF (R)				
% BODY FAT				

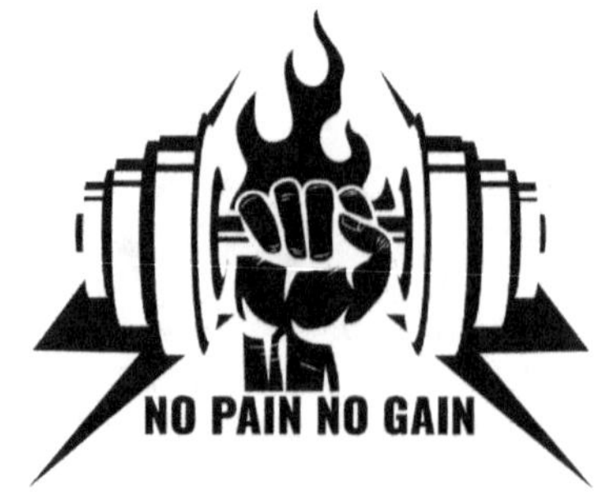

	DATE:_______	DATE:_______	DATE:_______	DATE:_______
WEIGHT				
NECK				
SHOULDERS				
CHEST				
BICEP (L)				
BICEP (R)				
WAIST				
HIPS				
THIGH (L)				
THIGH (R)				
CALF (L)				
CALF (R)				
% BODY FAT				

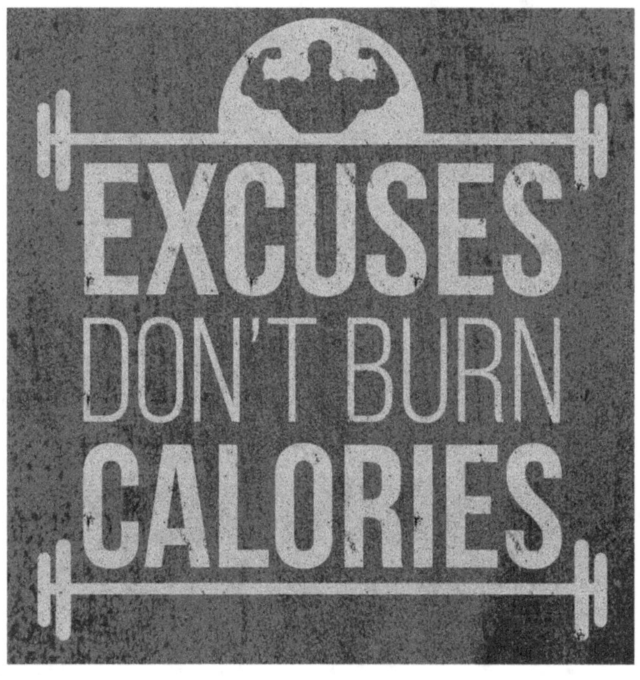

	DATE:______	DATE:______	DATE:______	DATE:______
WEIGHT				
NECK				
SHOULDERS				
CHEST				
BICEP (L)				
BICEP (R)				
WAIST				
HIPS				
THIGH (L)				
THIGH (R)				
CALF (L)				
CALF (R)				
% BODY FAT				

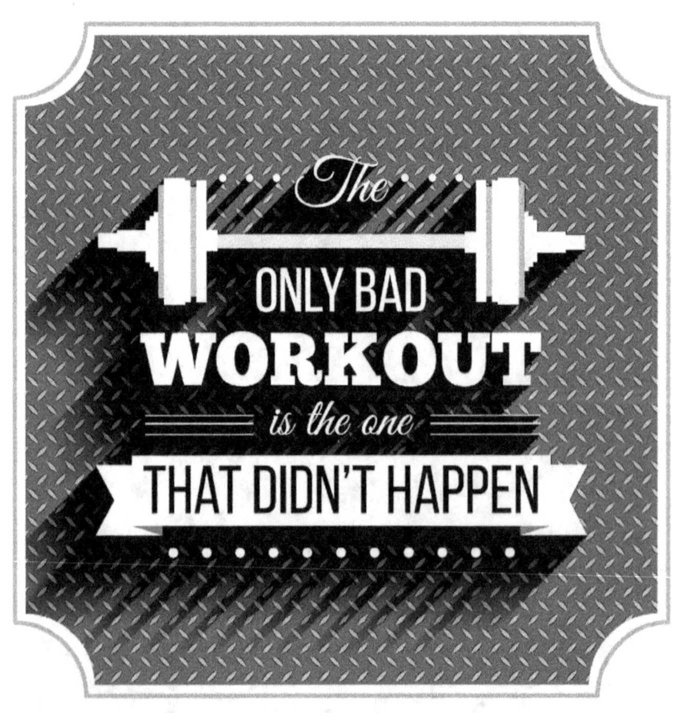

NUTRITION JOURNAL

DATE:	CALORIES	FAT	CARBS	WATER
MONDAY				
TUESDAY				
WEDNESDAY				
THURSDAY				
FRIDAY				
SATURDAY				
SUNDAY				

DATE:	CALORIES	FAT	CARBS	WATER
MONDAY				
TUESDAY				
WEDNESDAY				
THURSDAY				
FRIDAY				
SATURDAY				
SUNDAY				

DATE:	CALORIES	FAT	CARBS	WATER
MONDAY				
TUESDAY				
WEDNESDAY				
THURSDAY				
FRIDAY				
SATURDAY				
SUNDAY				

DATE:	CALORIES	FAT	CARBS	WATER
MONDAY				
TUESDAY				
WEDNESDAY				
THURSDAY				
FRIDAY				
SATURDAY				
SUNDAY				

DATE:	CALORIES	FAT	CARBS	WATER
MONDAY				
TUESDAY				
WEDNESDAY				
THURSDAY				
FRIDAY				
SATURDAY				
SUNDAY				

DATE:	CALORIES	FAT	CARBS	WATER
MONDAY				
TUESDAY				
WEDNESDAY				
THURSDAY				
FRIDAY				
SATURDAY				
SUNDAY				

DATE:	CALORIES	FAT	CARBS	WATER
MONDAY				
TUESDAY				
WEDNESDAY				
THURSDAY				
FRIDAY				
SATURDAY				
SUNDAY				

DATE:	CALORIES	FAT	CARBS	WATER
MONDAY				
TUESDAY				
WEDNESDAY				
THURSDAY				
FRIDAY				
SATURDAY				
SUNDAY				

DATE:	CALORIES	FAT	CARBS	WATER
MONDAY				
TUESDAY				
WEDNESDAY				
THURSDAY				
FRIDAY				
SATURDAY				
SUNDAY				

DATE:	CALORIES	FAT	CARBS	WATER
MONDAY				
TUESDAY				
WEDNESDAY				
THURSDAY				
FRIDAY				
SATURDAY				
SUNDAY				

DATE:	CALORIES	FAT	CARBS	WATER
MONDAY				
TUESDAY				
WEDNESDAY				
THURSDAY				
FRIDAY				
SATURDAY				
SUNDAY				

DATE:	CALORIES	FAT	CARBS	WATER
MONDAY				
TUESDAY				
WEDNESDAY				
THURSDAY				
FRIDAY				
SATURDAY				
SUNDAY				

DATE:	CALORIES	FAT	CARBS	WATER
MONDAY				
TUESDAY				
WEDNESDAY				
THURSDAY				
FRIDAY				
SATURDAY				
SUNDAY				

DATE:	CALORIES	FAT	CARBS	WATER
MONDAY				
TUESDAY				
WEDNESDAY				
THURSDAY				
FRIDAY				
SATURDAY				
SUNDAY				

DATE:	CALORIES	FAT	CARBS	WATER
MONDAY				
TUESDAY				
WEDNESDAY				
THURSDAY				
FRIDAY				
SATURDAY				
SUNDAY				

DATE:	CALORIES	FAT	CARBS	WATER
MONDAY				
TUESDAY				
WEDNESDAY				
THURSDAY				
FRIDAY				
SATURDAY				
SUNDAY				

DATE:	CALORIES	FAT	CARBS	WATER
MONDAY				
TUESDAY				
WEDNESDAY				
THURSDAY				
FRIDAY				
SATURDAY				
SUNDAY				

DATE:	CALORIES	FAT	CARBS	WATER
MONDAY				
TUESDAY				
WEDNESDAY				
THURSDAY				
FRIDAY				
SATURDAY				
SUNDAY				

DATE:	CALORIES	FAT	CARBS	WATER
MONDAY				
TUESDAY				
WEDNESDAY				
THURSDAY				
FRIDAY				
SATURDAY				
SUNDAY				

DATE:	CALORIES	FAT	CARBS	WATER
MONDAY				
TUESDAY				
WEDNESDAY				
THURSDAY				
FRIDAY				
SATURDAY				
SUNDAY				

DATE:	CALORIES	FAT	CARBS	WATER
MONDAY				
TUESDAY				
WEDNESDAY				
THURSDAY				
FRIDAY				
SATURDAY				
SUNDAY				

DATE:	CALORIES	FAT	CARBS	WATER
MONDAY				
TUESDAY				
WEDNESDAY				
THURSDAY				
FRIDAY				
SATURDAY				
SUNDAY				

DATE:	CALORIES	FAT	CARBS	WATER
MONDAY				
TUESDAY				
WEDNESDAY				
THURSDAY				
FRIDAY				
SATURDAY				
SUNDAY				

DATE:	CALORIES	FAT	CARBS	WATER
MONDAY				
TUESDAY				
WEDNESDAY				
THURSDAY				
FRIDAY				
SATURDAY				
SUNDAY				

DATE:	CALORIES	FAT	CARBS	WATER
MONDAY				
TUESDAY				
WEDNESDAY				
THURSDAY				
FRIDAY				
SATURDAY				
SUNDAY				

DATE:	CALORIES	FAT	CARBS	WATER
MONDAY				
TUESDAY				
WEDNESDAY				
THURSDAY				
FRIDAY				
SATURDAY				
SUNDAY				

DATE:	CALORIES	FAT	CARBS	WATER
MONDAY				
TUESDAY				
WEDNESDAY				
THURSDAY				
FRIDAY				
SATURDAY				
SUNDAY				

DATE:	CALORIES	FAT	CARBS	WATER
MONDAY				
TUESDAY				
WEDNESDAY				
THURSDAY				
FRIDAY				
SATURDAY				
SUNDAY				

DATE:	CALORIES	FAT	CARBS	WATER
MONDAY				
TUESDAY				
WEDNESDAY				
THURSDAY				
FRIDAY				
SATURDAY				
SUNDAY				

DATE:	CALORIES	FAT	CARBS	WATER
MONDAY				
TUESDAY				
WEDNESDAY				
THURSDAY				
FRIDAY				
SATURDAY				
SUNDAY				

DATE:	CALORIES	FAT	CARBS	WATER
MONDAY				
TUESDAY				
WEDNESDAY				
THURSDAY				
FRIDAY				
SATURDAY				
SUNDAY				

DATE:	CALORIES	FAT	CARBS	WATER
MONDAY				
TUESDAY				
WEDNESDAY				
THURSDAY				
FRIDAY				
SATURDAY				
SUNDAY				

DATE:	CALORIES	FAT	CARBS	WATER
MONDAY				
TUESDAY				
WEDNESDAY				
THURSDAY				
FRIDAY				
SATURDAY				
SUNDAY				

DATE:	CALORIES	FAT	CARBS	WATER
MONDAY				
TUESDAY				
WEDNESDAY				
THURSDAY				
FRIDAY				
SATURDAY				
SUNDAY				

DATE:	CALORIES	FAT	CARBS	WATER
MONDAY				
TUESDAY				
WEDNESDAY				
THURSDAY				
FRIDAY				
SATURDAY				
SUNDAY				

DATE:	CALORIES	FAT	CARBS	WATER
MONDAY				
TUESDAY				
WEDNESDAY				
THURSDAY				
FRIDAY				
SATURDAY				
SUNDAY				

DATE:	CALORIES	FAT	CARBS	WATER
MONDAY				
TUESDAY				
WEDNESDAY				
THURSDAY				
FRIDAY				
SATURDAY				
SUNDAY				

DATE:	CALORIES	FAT	CARBS	WATER
MONDAY				
TUESDAY				
WEDNESDAY				
THURSDAY				
FRIDAY				
SATURDAY				
SUNDAY				

DATE:	CALORIES	FAT	CARBS	WATER
MONDAY				
TUESDAY				
WEDNESDAY				
THURSDAY				
FRIDAY				
SATURDAY				
SUNDAY				

DATE:	CALORIES	FAT	CARBS	WATER
MONDAY				
TUESDAY				
WEDNESDAY				
THURSDAY				
FRIDAY				
SATURDAY				
SUNDAY				

DATE:	CALORIES	FAT	CARBS	WATER
MONDAY				
TUESDAY				
WEDNESDAY				
THURSDAY				
FRIDAY				
SATURDAY				
SUNDAY				

DATE:	CALORIES	FAT	CARBS	WATER
MONDAY				
TUESDAY				
WEDNESDAY				
THURSDAY				
FRIDAY				
SATURDAY				
SUNDAY				

DATE:	CALORIES	FAT	CARBS	WATER
MONDAY				
TUESDAY				
WEDNESDAY				
THURSDAY				
FRIDAY				
SATURDAY				
SUNDAY				

DATE:	CALORIES	FAT	CARBS	WATER
MONDAY				
TUESDAY				
WEDNESDAY				
THURSDAY				
FRIDAY				
SATURDAY				
SUNDAY				

DATE:	CALORIES	FAT	CARBS	WATER
MONDAY				
TUESDAY				
WEDNESDAY				
THURSDAY				
FRIDAY				
SATURDAY				
SUNDAY				

DATE:	CALORIES	FAT	CARBS	WATER
MONDAY				
TUESDAY				
WEDNESDAY				
THURSDAY				
FRIDAY				
SATURDAY				
SUNDAY				

DATE:	CALORIES	FAT	CARBS	WATER
MONDAY				
TUESDAY				
WEDNESDAY				
THURSDAY				
FRIDAY				
SATURDAY				
SUNDAY				

DATE:	CALORIES	FAT	CARBS	WATER
MONDAY				
TUESDAY				
WEDNESDAY				
THURSDAY				
FRIDAY				
SATURDAY				
SUNDAY				

DATE:	CALORIES	FAT	CARBS	WATER
MONDAY				
TUESDAY				
WEDNESDAY				
THURSDAY				
FRIDAY				
SATURDAY				
SUNDAY				

DATE:	CALORIES	FAT	CARBS	WATER
MONDAY				
TUESDAY				
WEDNESDAY				
THURSDAY				
FRIDAY				
SATURDAY				
SUNDAY				

DATE:	CALORIES	FAT	CARBS	WATER
MONDAY				
TUESDAY				
WEDNESDAY				
THURSDAY				
FRIDAY				
SATURDAY				
SUNDAY				

DATE:	CALORIES	FAT	CARBS	WATER
MONDAY				
TUESDAY				
WEDNESDAY				
THURSDAY				
FRIDAY				
SATURDAY				
SUNDAY				

DATE:	CALORIES	FAT	CARBS	WATER
MONDAY				
TUESDAY				
WEDNESDAY				
THURSDAY				
FRIDAY				
SATURDAY				
SUNDAY				

DATE:	CALORIES	FAT	CARBS	WATER
MONDAY				
TUESDAY				
WEDNESDAY				
THURSDAY				
FRIDAY				
SATURDAY				
SUNDAY				

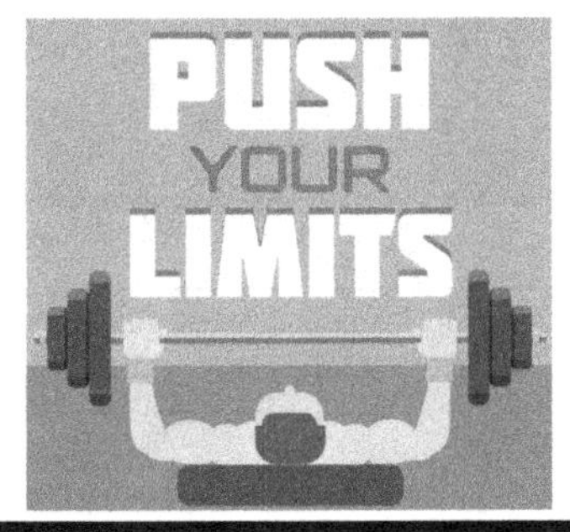

GOAL PAGES

DATE:			
EXERCISE			
EXAMPLE	REPS	10	
	WEIGHT	125 LBS	

NOTES

GOAL PAGES

DATE:			
EXERCISE			

NOTES

GOAL PAGES

DATE:			
EXERCISE			

"DO SOMETHING TODAY THAT YOUR FUTURE SELF WILL THANK YOU FOR."
-UNKNOWN

NOTES

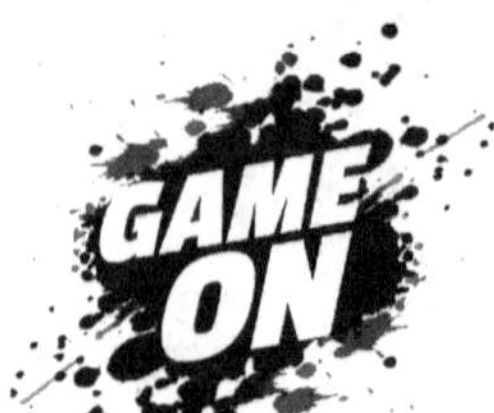

DAILY WORKOUT LOGS

DATE:	START TIME:			END TIME:		
EXERCISE	**Set 1**	**Set 2**	**Set 3**	**Set 4**	**Set 5**	**Set 6**
EXAMPLE	REPS	10				
	WEIGHT	125 LBS				

DATE:	START TIME:			END TIME:		
EXERCISE	Set 1	Set 2	Set 3	Set 4	Set 5	Set 6

NOTES

DATE:	START TIME:			END TIME:		
EXERCISE	Set 1	Set 2	Set 3	Set 4	Set 5	Set 6

NOTES

<table>
<tr><td>DATE:</td><td colspan="2">START TIME:</td><td colspan="2">END TIME:</td><td></td></tr>
</table>

EXERCISE	Set 1	Set 2	Set 3	Set 4	Set 5	Set 6

THE LAST THREE OR FOUR REPS IS WHAT MAKES THE MUSCLE GROW.
THIS AREA OF PAIN DIVIDES THE CHAMPION FROM SOMEONE ELSE
WHO IS NOT A CHAMPION.

-ARNOLD SCHWARZENEGGER

NOTES

DATE:	START TIME:			END TIME:		
EXERCISE	Set 1	Set 2	Set 3	Set 4	Set 5	Set 6

NOTES

| DATE: | START TIME: | | | END TIME: | | |
EXERCISE	Set 1	Set 2	Set 3	Set 4	Set 5	Set 6

NOTES

DATE:	START TIME:			END TIME:		
EXERCISE	**Set 1**	**Set 2**	**Set 3**	**Set 4**	**Set 5**	**Set 6**

NOTES

<table>
<tr><td>DATE:</td><td colspan="2">START TIME:</td><td colspan="4">END TIME:</td></tr>
</table>

EXERCISE	Set 1	Set 2	Set 3	Set 4	Set 5	Set 6

NOTES

<table>
<tr><td colspan="2">DATE:</td><td colspan="2">START TIME:</td><td colspan="3">END TIME:</td></tr>
<tr><td>EXERCISE</td><td>Set 1</td><td>Set 2</td><td>Set 3</td><td>Set 4</td><td>Set 5</td><td>Set 6</td></tr>
</table>

NOTES

| DATE: | START TIME: | | | END TIME: | | |
EXERCISE	Set 1	Set 2	Set 3	Set 4	Set 5	Set 6

"YOU HAVE TO PUSH PAST YOUR PERCEIVED LIMITS, PUSH PAST THAT POINT YOU THOUGHT WAS AS FAR AS YOU CAN GO."

-DREW BREES

NOTES

<table>
<tr><td>DATE:</td><td colspan="2">START TIME:</td><td colspan="4">END TIME:</td></tr>
<tr><td>EXERCISE</td><td>Set 1</td><td>Set 2</td><td>Set 3</td><td>Set 4</td><td>Set 5</td><td>Set 6</td></tr>
</table>

NOTES

DATE:	START TIME:			END TIME:		
EXERCISE	Set 1	Set 2	Set 3	Set 4	Set 5	Set 6

NOTES

DATE:	START TIME:			END TIME:		
EXERCISE	Set 1	Set 2	Set 3	Set 4	Set 5	Set 6

NOTES

DATE:	START TIME:			END TIME:		
EXERCISE	Set 1	Set 2	Set 3	Set 4	Set 5	Set 6

"REMEMBER THIS: YOUR BODY IS YOUR SLAVE; IT WORKS FOR YOU."
-JACK LALANNE

NOTES

DATE:	START TIME:			END TIME:		
EXERCISE	**Set 1**	**Set 2**	**Set 3**	**Set 4**	**Set 5**	**Set 6**

NOTES

<table>
<tr><td>DATE:</td><td colspan="3">START TIME:</td><td colspan="3">END TIME:</td></tr>
<tr><td>EXERCISE</td><td>Set 1</td><td>Set 2</td><td>Set 3</td><td>Set 4</td><td>Set 5</td><td>Set 6</td></tr>
</table>

NOTES

<table>
<tr><td colspan="7">DATE: START TIME: END TIME:</td></tr>
<tr><td>EXERCISE</td><td>Set 1</td><td>Set 2</td><td>Set 3</td><td>Set 4</td><td>Set 5</td><td>Set 6</td></tr>
</table>

NOTES

DATE:	START TIME:			END TIME:		
EXERCISE	Set 1	Set 2	Set 3	Set 4	Set 5	Set 6

"THE ONLY EASY DAY WAS YESTERDAY."

-NAVY SEALS

NOTES

DATE:	START TIME:			END TIME:		
EXERCISE	Set 1	Set 2	Set 3	Set 4	Set 5	Set 6

NOTES

DATE:	START TIME:			END TIME:		
EXERCISE	**Set 1**	**Set 2**	**Set 3**	**Set 4**	**Set 5**	**Set 6**

"YOU WANT ME TO DO SOMETHING… TELL ME I CAN'T DO IT."

-MAYA ANGELOU

NOTES

DATE:	START TIME:			END TIME:		
EXERCISE	Set 1	Set 2	Set 3	Set 4	Set 5	Set 6

NOTES

| DATE: | START TIME: | | | END TIME: | | |
EXERCISE	Set 1	Set 2	Set 3	Set 4	Set 5	Set 6

NOTES

DATE:	START TIME:			END TIME:		
EXERCISE	**Set 1**	**Set 2**	**Set 3**	**Set 4**	**Set 5**	**Set 6**

"AIN'T NUTTIN' TO IT, BUT TA DO IT."

-RONNIE COLEMAN

NOTES

DATE:	START TIME:			END TIME:		
EXERCISE	Set 1	Set 2	Set 3	Set 4	Set 5	Set 6

NOTES

<table>
<tr><td>DATE:</td><td colspan="2">START TIME:</td><td colspan="2">END TIME:</td><td></td></tr>
<tr><td>EXERCISE</td><td>Set 1</td><td>Set 2</td><td>Set 3</td><td>Set 4</td><td>Set 5</td><td>Set 6</td></tr>
</table>

NOTES

DATE:	START TIME:			END TIME:		
EXERCISE	Set 1	Set 2	Set 3	Set 4	Set 5	Set 6

NOTES

<table>
<tr><td>DATE:</td><td colspan="2">START TIME:</td><td colspan="2">END TIME:</td><td></td></tr>
<tr><td>EXERCISE</td><td>Set 1</td><td>Set 2</td><td>Set 3</td><td>Set 4</td><td>Set 5</td><td>Set 6</td></tr>
</table>

NOTES

DATE:	START TIME:			END TIME:		
EXERCISE	Set 1	Set 2	Set 3	Set 4	Set 5	Set 6

"THOSE WHO THINK THEY HAVE NO TIME FOR BODILY EXERCISE WILL SOONER OR LATER HAVE TO FIND TIME FOR ILLNESS."

-EDWARD STANLEY

NOTES

<table>
<tr><td>DATE:</td><td colspan="2">START TIME:</td><td colspan="2">END TIME:</td><td></td></tr>
<tr><td>EXERCISE</td><td>Set 1</td><td>Set 2</td><td>Set 3</td><td>Set 4</td><td>Set 5</td><td>Set 6</td></tr>
</table>

NOTES

<table>
<tr><td>DATE:</td><td colspan="3">START TIME:</td><td colspan="3">END TIME:</td></tr>
<tr><td>EXERCISE</td><td>Set 1</td><td>Set 2</td><td>Set 3</td><td>Set 4</td><td>Set 5</td><td>Set 6</td></tr>
</table>

NOTES

EXERCISE	Set 1	Set 2	Set 3	Set 4	Set 5	Set 6
DATE:	START TIME:			END TIME:		

NOTES

DATE:	START TIME:			END TIME:		
EXERCISE	Set 1	Set 2	Set 3	Set 4	Set 5	Set 6

NOTES

<table>
<tr><td>DATE:</td><td colspan="3">START TIME:</td><td colspan="3">END TIME:</td></tr>
<tr><td>EXERCISE</td><td>Set 1</td><td>Set 2</td><td>Set 3</td><td>Set 4</td><td>Set 5</td><td>Set 6</td></tr>
</table>

NOTES

DATE:	START TIME:			END TIME:		
EXERCISE	Set 1	Set 2	Set 3	Set 4	Set 5	Set 6

NOTES

DATE:	START TIME:			END TIME:		
EXERCISE	Set 1	Set 2	Set 3	Set 4	Set 5	Set 6

"INTENSITY BUILDS IMMENSITY."

-KEVIN LEVRONE

NOTES

DATE:	START TIME:			END TIME:		
EXERCISE	Set 1	Set 2	Set 3	Set 4	Set 5	Set 6

NOTES

<table>
<tr><td colspan="2">DATE: .</td><td colspan="3">START TIME:</td><td colspan="3">END TIME:</td></tr>
</table>

EXERCISE	Set 1	Set 2	Set 3	Set 4	Set 5	Set 6

NOTES

DATE:	START TIME:			END TIME:		
EXERCISE	Set 1	Set 2	Set 3	Set 4	Set 5	Set 6

NOTES

DATE:	START TIME:			END TIME:		
EXERCISE	Set 1	Set 2	Set 3	Set 4	Set 5	Set 6

NOTES

| DATE: | START TIME: | | | END TIME: | | |
EXERCISE	Set 1	Set 2	Set 3	Set 4	Set 5	Set 6

NOTES

DATE:	START TIME:			END TIME:		
EXERCISE	**Set 1**	**Set 2**	**Set 3**	**Set 4**	**Set 5**	**Set 6**

"DON'T ASK FOR A LIGHT LOAD, BUT RATHER A STRONG BACK."

-UNKNOWN

NOTES

| DATE: | START TIME: | | | END TIME: | | |
EXERCISE	Set 1	Set 2	Set 3	Set 4	Set 5	Set 6

NOTES

DATE:	START TIME:			END TIME:		
EXERCISE	Set 1	Set 2	Set 3	Set 4	Set 5	Set 6

NOTES

DATE:	START TIME:			END TIME:		
EXERCISE	**Set 1**	**Set 2**	**Set 3**	**Set 4**	**Set 5**	**Set 6**

NOTES

<table>
<tr><td>DATE:</td><td colspan="3">START TIME:</td><td colspan="3">END TIME:</td></tr>
<tr><td>EXERCISE</td><td>Set 1</td><td>Set 2</td><td>Set 3</td><td>Set 4</td><td>Set 5</td><td>Set 6</td></tr>
</table>

NOTES

DATE:	START TIME:			END TIME:		
EXERCISE	**Set 1**	**Set 2**	**Set 3**	**Set 4**	**Set 5**	**Set 6**

NOTES

DATE:	START TIME:			END TIME:		
EXERCISE	Set 1	Set 2	Set 3	Set 4	Set 5	Set 6

"THE PAIN YOU FEEL TODAY IS THE STRENGTH YOU'LL FEEL TOMORROW."

- UNKNOWN

NOTES

<table>
<tr><td>DATE:</td><td colspan="3">START TIME:</td><td colspan="3">END TIME:</td></tr>
<tr><td>EXERCISE</td><td>Set 1</td><td>Set 2</td><td>Set 3</td><td>Set 4</td><td>Set 5</td><td>Set 6</td></tr>
</table>

NOTES

DATE:	START TIME:			END TIME:		
EXERCISE	**Set 1**	**Set 2**	**Set 3**	**Set 4**	**Set 5**	**Set 6**

NOTES

DATE:	START TIME:			END TIME:		
EXERCISE	Set 1	Set 2	Set 3	Set 4	Set 5	Set 6

NOTES

<table>
<tr><td>DATE:</td><td colspan="3">START TIME:</td><td colspan="3">END TIME:</td></tr>
</table>

EXERCISE	Set 1	Set 2	Set 3	Set 4	Set 5	Set 6

NOTES

<table>
<tr><td>DATE:</td><td colspan="2">START TIME:</td><td colspan="3">END TIME:</td></tr>
<tr><td>EXERCISE</td><td>Set 1</td><td>Set 2</td><td>Set 3</td><td>Set 4</td><td>Set 5</td><td>Set 6</td></tr>
</table>

NOTES

DATE:	START TIME:			END TIME:		
EXERCISE	Set 1	Set 2	Set 3	Set 4	Set 5	Set 6

THE FIGHT IS WON OR LOST FAR AWAY FROM WITNESSES, BEHIND THE LINES, IN THE GYM…"

-MUHAMMAD ALI

NOTES

EXERCISE	Set 1	Set 2	Set 3	Set 4	Set 5	Set 6

NOTES

<table>
<tr><td>DATE:</td><td colspan="3">START TIME:</td><td colspan="3">END TIME:</td></tr>
<tr><td>EXERCISE</td><td>Set 1</td><td>Set 2</td><td>Set 3</td><td>Set 4</td><td>Set 5</td><td>Set 6</td></tr>
</table>

NOTES

<table>
<tr><td colspan="2">DATE:</td><td colspan="2">START TIME:</td><td colspan="3">END TIME:</td></tr>
<tr><td>EXERCISE</td><td>Set 1</td><td>Set 2</td><td>Set 3</td><td>Set 4</td><td>Set 5</td><td>Set 6</td></tr>
</table>

NOTES

DATE:	START TIME:			END TIME:		
EXERCISE	**Set 1**	**Set 2**	**Set 3**	**Set 4**	**Set 5**	**Set 6**

NOTES

| DATE: | START TIME: | | | END TIME: | | |
EXERCISE	Set 1	Set 2	Set 3	Set 4	Set 5	Set 6

NOTES

| DATE: | START TIME: | | | END TIME: | | |
EXERCISE	Set 1	Set 2	Set 3	Set 4	Set 5	Set 6

"TAKE CARE OF YOUR BODY. IT'S THE ONLY PLACE YOU HAVE TO LIVE."
- JIM ROHN

NOTES

<table>
<tr><td>DATE:</td><td colspan="3">START TIME:</td><td colspan="3">END TIME:</td></tr>
<tr><td>EXERCISE</td><td>Set 1</td><td>Set 2</td><td>Set 3</td><td>Set 4</td><td>Set 5</td><td>Set 6</td></tr>
</table>

NOTES

<table>
<tr><td>DATE:</td><td colspan="3">START TIME:</td><td colspan="3">END TIME:</td></tr>
<tr><td>EXERCISE</td><td>Set 1</td><td>Set 2</td><td>Set 3</td><td>Set 4</td><td>Set 5</td><td>Set 6</td></tr>
</table>

NOTES

DATE:	START TIME:			END TIME:		
EXERCISE	Set 1	Set 2	Set 3	Set 4	Set 5	Set 6

NOTES

DATE:	START TIME:			END TIME:		
EXERCISE	Set 1	Set 2	Set 3	Set 4	Set 5	Set 6

NOTES

DATE:	START TIME:			END TIME:		
EXERCISE	Set 1	Set 2	Set 3	Set 4	Set 5	Set 6

NOTES

DATE:	START TIME:			END TIME:		
EXERCISE	Set 1	Set 2	Set 3	Set 4	Set 5	Set 6

NOTES

DATE:	START TIME:			END TIME:		
EXERCISE	Set 1	Set 2	Set 3	Set 4	Set 5	Set 6

"EVERYBODY WANTS TO BE A BODYBUILDER, BUT DON'T NOBODY
WANNA LIFT NO HEAVY WEIGHT."

— RONNIE COLEMAN

NOTES

DATE:	START TIME:			END TIME:		
EXERCISE	**Set 1**	**Set 2**	**Set 3**	**Set 4**	**Set 5**	**Set 6**

NOTES

<table>
<tr><td>DATE:</td><td colspan="2">START TIME:</td><td colspan="2">END TIME:</td></tr>
<tr><td>EXERCISE</td><td>Set 1</td><td>Set 2</td><td>Set 3</td><td>Set 4</td><td>Set 5</td><td>Set 6</td></tr>
</table>

NOTES

<table>
<tr><td colspan="2">DATE:</td><td colspan="2">START TIME:</td><td colspan="3">END TIME:</td></tr>
<tr><td>EXERCISE</td><td>Set 1</td><td>Set 2</td><td>Set 3</td><td>Set 4</td><td>Set 5</td><td>Set 6</td></tr>
</table>

NOTES

| DATE: | START TIME: | | | END TIME: | | |
EXERCISE	Set 1	Set 2	Set 3	Set 4	Set 5	Set 6

NOTES

DATE:	START TIME:			END TIME:		
EXERCISE	Set 1	Set 2	Set 3	Set 4	Set 5	Set 6

NOTES

DATE:	START TIME:			END TIME:		
EXERCISE	Set 1	Set 2	Set 3	Set 4	Set 5	Set 6

"A MAN'S HEALTH CAN BE JUDGED BY WHICH HE TAKES TWO AT A TIME - PILLS OR STAIRS."

-JOAN WELSH

NOTES

<table>
<tr><td>DATE:</td><td colspan="2">START TIME:</td><td colspan="4">END TIME:</td></tr>
<tr><td>EXERCISE</td><td>Set 1</td><td>Set 2</td><td>Set 3</td><td>Set 4</td><td>Set 5</td><td>Set 6</td></tr>
</table>

NOTES

<table>
<tr><td>DATE:</td><td colspan="3">START TIME:</td><td colspan="3">END TIME:</td></tr>
</table>

EXERCISE	Set 1	Set 2	Set 3	Set 4	Set 5	Set 6

NOTES

| DATE: | START TIME: | | | END TIME: | | |
EXERCISE	Set 1	Set 2	Set 3	Set 4	Set 5	Set 6

NOTES

DATE:	START TIME:			END TIME:		
EXERCISE	Set 1	Set 2	Set 3	Set 4	Set 5	Set 6

NOTES

DATE:	START TIME:			END TIME:		
EXERCISE	Set 1	Set 2	Set 3	Set 4	Set 5	Set 6

NOTES

<table>
<tr><td>DATE:</td><td colspan="2">START TIME:</td><td colspan="3">END TIME:</td></tr>
<tr><td>EXERCISE</td><td>Set 1</td><td>Set 2</td><td>Set 3</td><td>Set 4</td><td>Set 5</td><td>Set 6</td></tr>
</table>

NOTES

DATE:	START TIME:			END TIME:		
EXERCISE	Set 1	Set 2	Set 3	Set 4	Set 5	Set 6

NOTES

DATE:	START TIME:			END TIME:		
EXERCISE	Set 1	Set 2	Set 3	Set 4	Set 5	Set 6

"IF YOU DON'T DO WHAT'S BEST FOR YOUR BODY, YOU'RE THE ONE WHO COMES UP ON THE SHORT END."

— JULIUS ERVING

NOTES

| DATE: | START TIME: | | | END TIME: | | |
EXERCISE	Set 1	Set 2	Set 3	Set 4	Set 5	Set 6

NOTES

DATE:	START TIME:			END TIME:		
EXERCISE	Set 1	Set 2	Set 3	Set 4	Set 5	Set 6

NOTES

DATE:	START TIME:			END TIME:		
EXERCISE	**Set 1**	**Set 2**	**Set 3**	**Set 4**	**Set 5**	**Set 6**

NOTES

DATE:	START TIME:			END TIME:		
EXERCISE	Set 1	Set 2	Set 3	Set 4	Set 5	Set 6

NOTES

DATE:	START TIME:			END TIME:		
EXERCISE	**Set 1**	**Set 2**	**Set 3**	**Set 4**	**Set 5**	**Set 6**

NOTES

DATE:	START TIME:			END TIME:		
EXERCISE	Set 1	Set 2	Set 3	Set 4	Set 5	Set 6

NOTES

DATE:	START TIME:			END TIME:		
EXERCISE	**Set 1**	**Set 2**	**Set 3**	**Set 4**	**Set 5**	**Set 6**

NOTES

DATE:	START TIME:			END TIME:		
EXERCISE	Set 1	Set 2	Set 3	Set 4	Set 5	Set 6

NOTES

DATE:	START TIME:			END TIME:		
EXERCISE	**Set 1**	**Set 2**	**Set 3**	**Set 4**	**Set 5**	**Set 6**

NOTES

DATE:	START TIME:			END TIME:		
EXERCISE	**Set 1**	**Set 2**	**Set 3**	**Set 4**	**Set 5**	**Set 6**

DATE:	START TIME:			END TIME:		
EXERCISE	Set 1	Set 2	Set 3	Set 4	Set 5	Set 6

"IF YOU'RE CAPABLE OF SENDING A LEGIBLE TEXT MESSAGE BETWEEN SETS, YOU PROBABLY AREN'T WORKING HARD ENOUGH."

— DAVE TATE

NOTES

DATE:	START TIME:			END TIME:		
EXERCISE	Set 1	Set 2	Set 3	Set 4	Set 5	Set 6

NOTES

DATE:	START TIME:			END TIME:		
EXERCISE	Set 1	Set 2	Set 3	Set 4	Set 5	Set 6

NOTES

<table>
<tr><td>DATE:</td><td colspan="3">START TIME:</td><td colspan="3">END TIME:</td></tr>
</table>

EXERCISE	Set 1	Set 2	Set 3	Set 4	Set 5	Set 6

NOTES

DATE:	START TIME:			END TIME:		
EXERCISE	Set 1	Set 2	Set 3	Set 4	Set 5	Set 6

NOTES

DATE:	START TIME:			END TIME:		
EXERCISE	Set 1	Set 2	Set 3	Set 4	Set 5	Set 6

NOTES

DATE:	START TIME:			END TIME:		
EXERCISE	**Set 1**	**Set 2**	**Set 3**	**Set 4**	**Set 5**	**Set 6**

NOTES

DATE:	START TIME:			END TIME:		
EXERCISE	Set 1	Set 2	Set 3	Set 4	Set 5	Set 6

"A CHAMPION IS SOMEONE WHO GETS UP WHEN THEY CAN'T."

— JACK DEMPSEY

DATE:	START TIME:			END TIME:		
EXERCISE	Set 1	Set 2	Set 3	Set 4	Set 5	Set 6

NOTES

<table>
<tr><td colspan="1">DATE:</td><td colspan="2">START TIME:</td><td colspan="2">END TIME:</td><td></td></tr>
<tr><td>EXERCISE</td><td>Set 1</td><td>Set 2</td><td>Set 3</td><td>Set 4</td><td>Set 5</td><td>Set 6</td></tr>
</table>

NOTES

DATE:	START TIME:			END TIME:		
EXERCISE	**Set 1**	**Set 2**	**Set 3**	**Set 4**	**Set 5**	**Set 6**

NOTES

| DATE: | START TIME: | | | END TIME: | | |
EXERCISE	Set 1	Set 2	Set 3	Set 4	Set 5	Set 6

NOTES

<table>
<tr><td>DATE:</td><td colspan="3">START TIME:</td><td colspan="3">END TIME:</td></tr>
<tr><td>EXERCISE</td><td>Set 1</td><td>Set 2</td><td>Set 3</td><td>Set 4</td><td>Set 5</td><td>Set 6</td></tr>
</table>

NOTES

DATE:	START TIME:			END TIME:		
EXERCISE	Set 1	Set 2	Set 3	Set 4	Set 5	Set 6

NOTES

DATE:	START TIME:			END TIME:		
EXERCISE	**Set 1**	**Set 2**	**Set 3**	**Set 4**	**Set 5**	**Set 6**

NOTES

EXERCISE	Set 1	Set 2	Set 3	Set 4	Set 5	Set 6
DATE:	START TIME:			END TIME:		

NOTES

| DATE: | START TIME: | | | END TIME: | | |
EXERCISE	Set 1	Set 2	Set 3	Set 4	Set 5	Set 6

NOTES

DATE:	START TIME:			END TIME:		
EXERCISE	Set 1	Set 2	Set 3	Set 4	Set 5	Set 6

"THE ROAD TO NOWHERE IS PAVED WITH EXCUSES."

– MARK BELL

<table>
<tr><td colspan="1">DATE:</td><td colspan="2">START TIME:</td><td colspan="3">END TIME:</td></tr>
<tr><td>EXERCISE</td><td>Set 1</td><td>Set 2</td><td>Set 3</td><td>Set 4</td><td>Set 5</td><td>Set 6</td></tr>
</table>

NOTES

<table>
<tr><td>DATE:</td><td colspan="3">START TIME:</td><td colspan="3">END TIME:</td></tr>
<tr><td>EXERCISE</td><td>Set 1</td><td>Set 2</td><td>Set 3</td><td>Set 4</td><td>Set 5</td><td>Set 6</td></tr>
</table>

NOTES

DATE:	START TIME:			END TIME:		
EXERCISE	Set 1	Set 2	Set 3	Set 4	Set 5	Set 6

NOTES

DATE:	START TIME:			END TIME:		
EXERCISE	Set 1	Set 2	Set 3	Set 4	Set 5	Set 6

NOTES

<table>
<tr><td>DATE:</td><td colspan="2">START TIME:</td><td colspan="2">END TIME:</td><td></td></tr>
<tr><td>EXERCISE</td><td>Set 1</td><td>Set 2</td><td>Set 3</td><td>Set 4</td><td>Set 5</td><td>Set 6</td></tr>
</table>

NOTES

DATE:	START TIME:			END TIME:		
EXERCISE	Set 1	Set 2	Set 3	Set 4	Set 5	Set 6

NOTES

<table>
<tr><td>DATE:</td><td colspan="3">START TIME:</td><td colspan="3">END TIME:</td></tr>
<tr><td>EXERCISE</td><td>Set 1</td><td>Set 2</td><td>Set 3</td><td>Set 4</td><td>Set 5</td><td>Set 6</td></tr>
</table>

NOTES

DATE:	START TIME:			END TIME:		
EXERCISE	**Set 1**	**Set 2**	**Set 3**	**Set 4**	**Set 5**	**Set 6**

NOTES

DATE:	START TIME:			END TIME:		
EXERCISE	Set 1	Set 2	Set 3	Set 4	Set 5	Set 6

NOTES

DATE:	START TIME:			END TIME:		
EXERCISE	**Set 1**	**Set 2**	**Set 3**	**Set 4**	**Set 5**	**Set 6**

NOTES

DATE:	START TIME:			END TIME:		
EXERCISE	Set 1	Set 2	Set 3	Set 4	Set 5	Set 6

"THERE'S MORE TO LIFE THAN TRAINING, BUT TRAINING IS WHAT PUTS MORE IN YOUR LIFE."

— BROOKS KUBIK

NOTES

<table>
<tr><td>DATE:</td><td colspan="3">START TIME:</td><td colspan="3">END TIME:</td></tr>
<tr><td>EXERCISE</td><td>Set 1</td><td>Set 2</td><td>Set 3</td><td>Set 4</td><td>Set 5</td><td>Set 6</td></tr>
</table>

NOTES

<table>
<tr><td>DATE:</td><td colspan="2">START TIME:</td><td colspan="4">END TIME:</td></tr>
<tr><td>EXERCISE</td><td>Set 1</td><td>Set 2</td><td>Set 3</td><td>Set 4</td><td>Set 5</td><td>Set 6</td></tr>
</table>

NOTES

<table>
<tr><td colspan="1">DATE:</td><td colspan="2">START TIME:</td><td colspan="3">END TIME:</td></tr>
<tr><td>EXERCISE</td><td>Set 1</td><td>Set 2</td><td>Set 3</td><td>Set 4</td><td>Set 5</td><td>Set 6</td></tr>
</table>

NOTES

DATE:	START TIME:			END TIME:		
EXERCISE	Set 1	Set 2	Set 3	Set 4	Set 5	Set 6

NOTES

| DATE: | START TIME: | | | END TIME: | | |
EXERCISE	Set 1	Set 2	Set 3	Set 4	Set 5	Set 6

NOTES

DATE:	START TIME:			END TIME:		
EXERCISE	Set 1	Set 2	Set 3	Set 4	Set 5	Set 6

NOTES

<table>
<tr><td>DATE:</td><td colspan="2">START TIME:</td><td colspan="2">END TIME:</td></tr>
<tr><td>EXERCISE</td><td>Set 1</td><td>Set 2</td><td>Set 3</td><td>Set 4</td><td>Set 5</td><td>Set 6</td></tr>
</table>

NOTES

<table>
<tr><td>DATE:</td><td colspan="2">START TIME:</td><td colspan="2">END TIME:</td></tr>
<tr><td>EXERCISE</td><td>Set 1</td><td>Set 2</td><td>Set 3</td><td>Set 4</td><td>Set 5</td><td>Set 6</td></tr>
</table>

DATE:	START TIME:			END TIME:		
EXERCISE	**Set 1**	**Set 2**	**Set 3**	**Set 4**	**Set 5**	**Set 6**

NOTES

<table>
<tr><td>DATE:</td><td colspan="2">START TIME:</td><td colspan="4">END TIME:</td></tr>
<tr><td>EXERCISE</td><td>Set 1</td><td>Set 2</td><td>Set 3</td><td>Set 4</td><td>Set 5</td><td>Set 6</td></tr>
</table>

NOTES

DATE:	START TIME:			END TIME:		
EXERCISE	**Set 1**	**Set 2**	**Set 3**	**Set 4**	**Set 5**	**Set 6**

NOTES

DATE:	START TIME:			END TIME:		
EXERCISE	Set 1	Set 2	Set 3	Set 4	Set 5	Set 6

"I NEVER THINK ABOUT LOSING."

\- LOU FERRIGNO

NOTES

DATE:	START TIME:			END TIME:		
EXERCISE	Set 1	Set 2	Set 3	Set 4	Set 5	Set 6

NOTES

DATE:	START TIME:			END TIME:		
EXERCISE	Set 1	Set 2	Set 3	Set 4	Set 5	Set 6

NOTES

DATE:	START TIME:			END TIME:		
EXERCISE	Set 1	Set 2	Set 3	Set 4	Set 5	Set 6

NOTES

| DATE: | START TIME: | | | END TIME: | | |
EXERCISE	Set 1	Set 2	Set 3	Set 4	Set 5	Set 6

NOTES

| DATE: | START TIME: | | | END TIME: | | |
EXERCISE	Set 1	Set 2	Set 3	Set 4	Set 5	Set 6

NOTES

| DATE: | START TIME: | | | END TIME: | | |
EXERCISE	Set 1	Set 2	Set 3	Set 4	Set 5	Set 6

NOTES

EXERCISE	Set 1	Set 2	Set 3	Set 4	Set 5	Set 6

NOTES

DATE:	START TIME:			END TIME:		
EXERCISE	Set 1	Set 2	Set 3	Set 4	Set 5	Set 6

NOTES

DATE:	START TIME:			END TIME:		
EXERCISE	Set 1	Set 2	Set 3	Set 4	Set 5	Set 6

NOTES

DATE:	START TIME:			END TIME:		
EXERCISE	**Set 1**	**Set 2**	**Set 3**	**Set 4**	**Set 5**	**Set 6**

"COURAGE DOESN'T ALWAYS ROAR. SOMETIMES COURAGE IS THE QUIET VOICE AT THE END OF THE DAY SAYING, 'I WILL TRY AGAIN TOMORROW.'"

- MARY ANNE RADMACHER

NOTES

DATE:	START TIME:			END TIME:		
EXERCISE	Set 1	Set 2	Set 3	Set 4	Set 5	Set 6

NOTES

DATE:	START TIME:			END TIME:		
EXERCISE	**Set 1**	**Set 2**	**Set 3**	**Set 4**	**Set 5**	**Set 6**

NOTES

<table>
<tr><td>DATE:</td><td colspan="3">START TIME:</td><td colspan="3">END TIME:</td></tr>
<tr><td>EXERCISE</td><td>Set 1</td><td>Set 2</td><td>Set 3</td><td>Set 4</td><td>Set 5</td><td>Set 6</td></tr>
</table>

NOTES

DATE:	START TIME:			END TIME:		
EXERCISE	Set 1	Set 2	Set 3	Set 4	Set 5	Set 6

NOTES

DATE:	START TIME:			END TIME:		
EXERCISE	Set 1	Set 2	Set 3	Set 4	Set 5	Set 6

NOTES

DATE:	START TIME:			END TIME:		
EXERCISE	Set 1	Set 2	Set 3	Set 4	Set 5	Set 6

NOTES

DATE:	START TIME:			END TIME:		
EXERCISE	Set 1	Set 2	Set 3	Set 4	Set 5	Set 6

NOTES

| DATE: | START TIME: | | | END TIME: | | |
EXERCISE	Set 1	Set 2	Set 3	Set 4	Set 5	Set 6

NOTES

DATE:	START TIME:			END TIME:		
EXERCISE	Set 1	Set 2	Set 3	Set 4	Set 5	Set 6

NOTES

DATE:	START TIME:			END TIME:		
EXERCISE	Set 1	Set 2	Set 3	Set 4	Set 5	Set 6

NOTES

| DATE: | START TIME: | | | END TIME: | | |
EXERCISE	Set 1	Set 2	Set 3	Set 4	Set 5	Set 6

NOTES

<table>
<tr><td>DATE:</td><td colspan="3">START TIME:</td><td colspan="3">END TIME:</td></tr>
<tr><td>EXERCISE</td><td>Set 1</td><td>Set 2</td><td>Set 3</td><td>Set 4</td><td>Set 5</td><td>Set 6</td></tr>
</table>

NOTES

DATE:	START TIME:			END TIME:		
EXERCISE	Set 1	Set 2	Set 3	Set 4	Set 5	Set 6

"DON'T GIVE UP WHAT YOU WANT MOST FOR WHAT YOU WANT NOW."

NOTES

DATE:	START TIME:			END TIME:		
EXERCISE	Set 1	Set 2	Set 3	Set 4	Set 5	Set 6

NOTES

DATE:	START TIME:			END TIME:		
EXERCISE	Set 1	Set 2	Set 3	Set 4	Set 5	Set 6

NOTES

| DATE: | START TIME: | | | END TIME: | | |
EXERCISE	Set 1	Set 2	Set 3	Set 4	Set 5	Set 6

NOTES

DATE:	START TIME:			END TIME:		
EXERCISE	Set 1	Set 2	Set 3	Set 4	Set 5	Set 6

NOTES

<table>
<tr><td>DATE:</td><td colspan="2">START TIME:</td><td colspan="4">END TIME:</td></tr>
<tr><td>EXERCISE</td><td>Set 1</td><td>Set 2</td><td>Set 3</td><td>Set 4</td><td>Set 5</td><td>Set 6</td></tr>
</table>

NOTES

DATE:	START TIME:			END TIME:		
EXERCISE	**Set 1**	**Set 2**	**Set 3**	**Set 4**	**Set 5**	**Set 6**

NOTES

DATE:	START TIME:			END TIME:		
EXERCISE	Set 1	Set 2	Set 3	Set 4	Set 5	Set 6

NOTES

DATE:	START TIME:			END TIME:		
EXERCISE	Set 1	Set 2	Set 3	Set 4	Set 5	Set 6

NOTES

DATE:	START TIME:			END TIME:		
EXERCISE	Set 1	Set 2	Set 3	Set 4	Set 5	Set 6

NOTES

DATE:	START TIME:			END TIME:		
EXERCISE	Set 1	Set 2	Set 3	Set 4	Set 5	Set 6

NOTES

DATE:	START TIME:			END TIME:		
EXERCISE	Set 1	Set 2	Set 3	Set 4	Set 5	Set 6

"DREAMS DON'T WORK UNLESS YOU DO."

NOTES

DATE:	START TIME:			END TIME:		
EXERCISE	Set 1	Set 2	Set 3	Set 4	Set 5	Set 6

NOTES

DATE:	START TIME:			END TIME:		
EXERCISE	Set 1	Set 2	Set 3	Set 4	Set 5	Set 6

NOTES

DATE:	START TIME:			END TIME:		
EXERCISE	Set 1	Set 2	Set 3	Set 4	Set 5	Set 6

NOTES

DATE:	START TIME:			END TIME:		
EXERCISE	Set 1	Set 2	Set 3	Set 4	Set 5	Set 6

NOTES

DATE:	START TIME:			END TIME:		
EXERCISE	Set 1	Set 2	Set 3	Set 4	Set 5	Set 6

NOTES

DATE:	START TIME:			END TIME:		
EXERCISE	Set 1	Set 2	Set 3	Set 4	Set 5	Set 6

NOTES

<table>
<tr><td>DATE:</td><td colspan="3">START TIME:</td><td colspan="3">END TIME:</td></tr>
<tr><td>EXERCISE</td><td>Set 1</td><td>Set 2</td><td>Set 3</td><td>Set 4</td><td>Set 5</td><td>Set 6</td></tr>
</table>

NOTES

<table>
<tr><td colspan="2">DATE:</td><td colspan="3">START TIME:</td><td colspan="2">END TIME:</td></tr>
</table>

EXERCISE	Set 1	Set 2	Set 3	Set 4	Set 5	Set 6

NOTES

DATE:	START TIME:			END TIME:		
EXERCISE	Set 1	Set 2	Set 3	Set 4	Set 5	Set 6

NOTES

DATE:	START TIME:			END TIME:		
EXERCISE	**Set 1**	**Set 2**	**Set 3**	**Set 4**	**Set 5**	**Set 6**

"IF IT DOESN'T CHALLENGE YOU, IT DOESN'T CHANGE YOU."

— FRED DEVITO

NOTES

DATE:	START TIME:			END TIME:		
EXERCISE	Set 1	Set 2	Set 3	Set 4	Set 5	Set 6

NOTES

DATE:	START TIME:			END TIME:		
EXERCISE	Set 1	Set 2	Set 3	Set 4	Set 5	Set 6

NOTES

DATE:	START TIME:			END TIME:		
EXERCISE	Set 1	Set 2	Set 3	Set 4	Set 5	Set 6

NOTES

DATE:	START TIME:			END TIME:		
EXERCISE	**Set 1**	**Set 2**	**Set 3**	**Set 4**	**Set 5**	**Set 6**

NOTES

<table>
<tr><td>DATE:</td><td colspan="2">START TIME:</td><td colspan="3">END TIME:</td></tr>
<tr><td>EXERCISE</td><td>Set 1</td><td>Set 2</td><td>Set 3</td><td>Set 4</td><td>Set 5</td><td>Set 6</td></tr>
</table>

NOTES

DATE:	START TIME:			END TIME:		
EXERCISE	Set 1	Set 2	Set 3	Set 4	Set 5	Set 6

NOTES

<table>
<tr><td>DATE:</td><td colspan="2">START TIME:</td><td colspan="4">END TIME:</td></tr>
<tr><td>EXERCISE</td><td>Set 1</td><td>Set 2</td><td>Set 3</td><td>Set 4</td><td>Set 5</td><td>Set 6</td></tr>
</table>

NOTES

DATE:	START TIME:			END TIME:		
EXERCISE	Set 1	Set 2	Set 3	Set 4	Set 5	Set 6

NOTES

DATE:	START TIME:			END TIME:		
EXERCISE	Set 1	Set 2	Set 3	Set 4	Set 5	Set 6

NOTES

DATE:	START TIME:			END TIME:		
EXERCISE	**Set 1**	**Set 2**	**Set 3**	**Set 4**	**Set 5**	**Set 6**

MOTIVATION IS WHAT GETS YOU STARTED. HABIT IS WHAT KEEPS YOU GOING."

— JIM RYAN

NOTES

<table>
<tr><td>DATE:</td><td colspan="3">START TIME:</td><td colspan="3">END TIME:</td></tr>
<tr><td>EXERCISE</td><td>Set 1</td><td>Set 2</td><td>Set 3</td><td>Set 4</td><td>Set 5</td><td>Set 6</td></tr>
</table>

NOTES

DATE:	START TIME:			END TIME:		
EXERCISE	Set 1	Set 2	Set 3	Set 4	Set 5	Set 6

NOTES

<table>
<tr><td colspan="1">DATE:</td><td colspan="3">START TIME:</td><td colspan="3">END TIME:</td></tr>
<tr><td>EXERCISE</td><td>Set 1</td><td>Set 2</td><td>Set 3</td><td>Set 4</td><td>Set 5</td><td>Set 6</td></tr>
</table>

NOTES

DATE:	START TIME:			END TIME:		
EXERCISE	Set 1	Set 2	Set 3	Set 4	Set 5	Set 6

NOTES

DATE:	START TIME:			END TIME:		
EXERCISE	Set 1	Set 2	Set 3	Set 4	Set 5	Set 6

NOTES

<table>
<tr><td>DATE:</td><td colspan="3">START TIME:</td><td colspan="3">END TIME:</td></tr>
<tr><td>EXERCISE</td><td>Set 1</td><td>Set 2</td><td>Set 3</td><td>Set 4</td><td>Set 5</td><td>Set 6</td></tr>
</table>

NOTES

EXERCISE	Set 1	Set 2	Set 3	Set 4	Set 5	Set 6

NOTES

<table>
<tr><td>DATE:</td><td colspan="3">START TIME:</td><td colspan="3">END TIME:</td></tr>
<tr><td>EXERCISE</td><td>Set 1</td><td>Set 2</td><td>Set 3</td><td>Set 4</td><td>Set 5</td><td>Set 6</td></tr>
</table>

NOTES

DATE:	START TIME:			END TIME:		
EXERCISE	Set 1	Set 2	Set 3	Set 4	Set 5	Set 6

NOTES

DATE:	START TIME:			END TIME:		
EXERCISE	Set 1	Set 2	Set 3	Set 4	Set 5	Set 6

NOTES

www.ingramcontent.com/pod-product-compliance
Lightning Source LLC
Chambersburg PA
CBHW071212240726
48654CB00009B/749